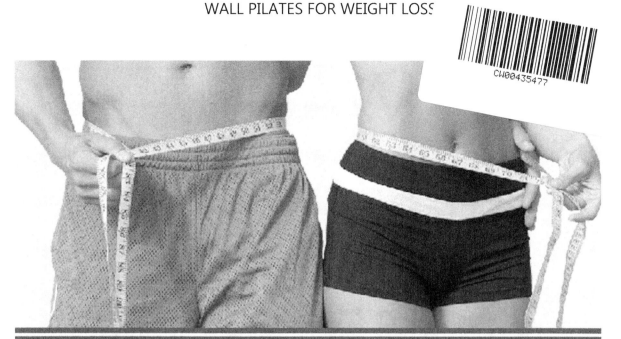

WALL PILATES FOR

WEIGHT LOSS

Quick and Effective Workout Routines for Maximum Weight Loss Suitable For Women and Seniors Over 60 With Step by Step Instructions and Visual Illustrations

RENEE J. HURT

WALL PILATES FOR WEIGHT LOSS

Quick and Effective Workout Routines for Maximum Weight Loss Suitable For Women and Seniors Over 60 With Step by Step Instructions and Visual Illustrations

Renee J. Hurt

OTHER BOOKS BY THE AUTHOR

2-MINS WALL PILATES FOR SENIORS

Scan below to get a COPY now

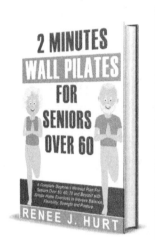 

2 MINUTES HOME WORKOUTS FOR SENIORS OVER 50

Scan below to get a COPY now

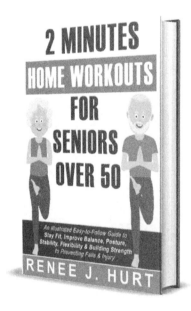 

CONTENT

WALL PILATES FOR WEIGHT LOSS

WALL PILATES FOR WEIGHT LOSS

INTRODUCTION

How many lies have you heard about weight loss? Quite a lot, I can imagine. Well, right off the bat, I can give you one of them for free. You would most likely have heard that" a radical exercise regime is the only way to lose weight." This is not true! For the average person, the thought of this automatically debilitates you. The good news, however, is that this statement is not exactly true. You need not be a Usain Bolt to lose weight.

The basic truth about weight loss is that you'll need to burn more calories than you consume to lose weight. How to go about this is a different story altogether; a radical exercise regime is not the only way to burn calories. A milder form of workout presents an alternative to the existing rigorous forms of exercising. If you've been very attentive recently, you must have heard of Pilates exercises. Originally called "controllogy" by founder Joseph Pilates, this form of workout has been practiced for over 90 years. The model is unique because it employs controlled movements to tone your body, enhance your posture, increase flexibility, and at the same time strengthens your abdominal muscles, most of which are vital for weight loss.

The beautiful thing about Pilates is that it stands in contrast to other highly physical exercising patterns; Pilates is a low-impact form of workout, allowing for gradual progress. However, conducting a regular Pilates routine usually requires specialized equipment like a Cadillac, wunda chair, or a reformer. The obvious implication of this is that unless you are ready to invest in this equipment or have access to a studio, it would appear that Pilates is not an alternative for you. Quite the contrary, you don't have to fret as there's a way to benefit from Pilates even without investing heavily.

Wall Pilates is the answer! This book introduces to you a very practicable technique for reaching your weight loss goals. If you are looking for a less daunting way of keeping fit, this book is made especially for you. It brings to you everything you need to know about using wall Pilates (a unique form of Pilates that uses a wall to aid and assist in exercising) to achieve your weight loss goals. This variation is a modified form of Pilates that uses a wall or any other suitable surface as support and resistance, making the exercise safe and effective while reducing the risk of injury.

Beyond uncovering popular myths about weight loss, this book will show you how you can get the best for yourself even without leaving the comfort of your home. Wall Pilates for weight loss is a book for you if you've often been terrified about the arduous nature of weight loss exercises. This book presents to you the ideal methods for using wall Pilates to achieve your weight loss goals, unearthing to you the precise methods and exercises that are perfect for burning calories.

Find out how you can use wall Pilates to lose weight, tone up, and create healthy and strong well-being from the inside out. From simplifying the exercises for beginners and strengthening the options for those who intend for a more challenging workout, Wall Pilates for weight loss is open to anybody who is intentional about changing their body build.

CHAPTER 1

WHAT IS WALL PILATES

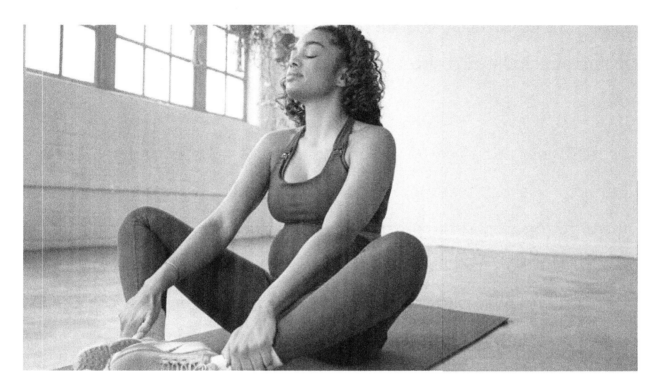

I invented all these machines... it resists your movements in just the right way, so those inner muscles really have to work against it. That way you can concentrate on movement. You must always do it slowly and smoothly. Then your whole body is in it. - Joseph Pilates.

Origin of Pilates

It is true that most obstacles in life end up becoming a step up. Pilates seems to be the talk of the time now; however, little or nothing would have been known about this practice if not for the resilience of Joseph Pilates. Exercises is mostly linked to the man Joseph Pilates, born in Dusseldorf, Germany, in 1883. He battled asthma, rickets, and Rheumatic fever; having a strong desire to overcome these ailments, he moved into the world of gymnastics and would also later become involved in sports like skiing and diving.

In 1912, Joseph moved to England to work as a boxer and self-defense instructor. He was later moved to intern with other German nationals, and there, he developed his physical fitness techniques. While serving as an orderly in a hospital where he assisted patients with difficulty walking, he attached bed springs to their limbs to help support them. This practice led to the development of the famous Cadillac.

Joseph and his wife Clara moved to the United States in the early 1920s; they taught this technique there in their body conditioning gym in New York. In the following years, Pilates wrote two materials on this topic: "your health" and "Return to health through controllogy." Through these books and his students, the practice has been passed down.

The Core Principles of Pilates

Grasping the basics of any subject is always critical to performing highly in that area. Though the originator was more a man of action than of theory, he founded this exercise on ideas that serve more or less like a structure. These eight principles of Pilates explain the philosophy behind this practice. Joseph Pilates based his work on three principles: Breath, whole-body health, and whole-body commitment. Though the principles are mostly categorized as being eight in number. He used the whole body to encompass mind, body, and spirit. It is through honoring these Pilate Principles that the depth of the work was achieved.

These fundamental principles are traditionally cited as follows:

1. Breath

2. Control

3. Precision

4. Center

5. Routine

6. Precision

7. Fluidity and

8. Isolation

If you can grasp these principles, your Pilates journey is sure to take a shorter period.

Concentration

Joseph believed that any exercise carried out without engaging the brain is no exercise at all. This led him to place key emphasis on the element of concentration. This element is at the heart of the Pilates philosophy. Take away focus, and nothing remains of Pilates. Unity between mind and body is vital to performing any Pilates exercise. Simply put, when in a Pilates' session, you must ensure you are in the most relaxed state possible, doing everything to avoid distraction.

Control

This notion for Pilate is not far from the everyday interpretation of control. The brain controls every limb, locomotion, or activity. In fact, every action in the body is linked to the brain. As one of the principles of Pilates, control explains the necessity of using the brain to instruct the muscles on what movement to perform, the varying intensity levels, and the particular extent of these movements.

If you're just starting out in Pilates, perfecting this exercise may be challenging, but continuous practice would put you on point.

Center

Often referred to by him as the powerhouse, Pilates believed the center of the body controls other movements in the body. This exercise regime stands in contrast to others like pushing, kicking, and running which focuses on extremities. Joseph Pilates believed that the center of the body is the point from which all movement is generated. He explained this point by giving an analogy of how ripples in a pond are formed from the center and then to the edges.

Having a strong center is crucial for the functioning of other parts of the body. Modern research has found that Pilates was accurate with his idea, the center houses so many muscles like those of the abdomen, lumbar, spine, and hips, and these muscles usually have multiple functions important to the functioning of the whole body.

Breathing

Breath control and breathing are essential parts of Pilate exercises. The originator often bothered that most people only breathed with the upper parts of their chest. This pattern of breathing, he thought, affects the precision of the movements needed and almost always makes it hard to complete the Pilates movement correctly. Instead, a pattern of breathing that entirely inflates the lungs with new air is preferable.

Lateral breathing is the style of breathing Pilates advocated for. Instead of raising the rib cage to inhale, please focus on the abdomen and lower ribcage muscles while trying to expand them outward. This more relaxed and controlled approach to breathing is essential to performing Pilates exercises.

Fluidity

Transitions from one exercise to the other in Pilates are meant to be seamless. Fluidity is the word Pilates used to describe flow in the different movements. He meant that the exercises and repetitions form part of one continuous exercise. In this light, there should be no one of them slower or the other faster; the intensity, speed, and distance moved should all be the same.

Precision

Every repetition in a Pilates exercise must be strictly the same, this is vital to making the overall process effective. Though digesting this principle would require your time and concentration, a Pilates exercise void of precision is compromised. Using a mirror and a sharp sense of visualization are great ways to help check progress while mastering precision.

Routine

This principle is akin to performing repetitions of most exercise routines. It is an indispensable way through which the muscles learn. A routine would ideally employ different methods of isolation to give us the balanced body Pilates builds for us.

Isolation

While other forms of exercising focus on isolating a particular set of muscles and then exercising them to tiredness, Pilates Isolation is usually made to be the introductory part of the exercise. In this way, Pilates used Isolation as the primary step to integration.

Wall Pilates Explained

The hard way is the only way, quite fine, but isn't it true that things can get better? Most people think of working out as a very tedious process that involves waking up every morning, leaving the house like you're late for school, and coming back home to think about the next day. If you're not a fan of this kind of setup, it becomes distressing to learn that Pilates doesn't appear to be the most practicable home workout. A traditional Pilates' routine would typically require having a studio, especially to give access to the specialized tools necessary to conduct a Pilates' exercise.

This is where wall Pilates comes in. Wall Pilates is a reformer-based Pilate exercise that uses your body weight with a wall that serves as a resistance to tone your muscles and improve your flexibility. The exercises in Pilates are slow and controlled, making this pattern of exercise ideal for persons new to Pilates. The low-impact nature of this workout makes it more suitable for beginners. The Good news about Wall Pilates is that all you need is a Wall. You heard that! You'd not have to bother about all of the equipment required in a regular Pilate routine. If you've ever worried about getting specialized training tools, Wall Pilates creates an opportunity for you.

This equipment, like a reformer and Cadillac, is mostly found in Pilates studios, but with Wall Pilates, all you need is a wall, and you can enjoy the benefits of regular Pilates exercise.

The Wall in Pilates helps give support and stamina to the individual new to Pilates. With this support, you are provided a feeling of security which helps ease the body into more demanding positions. If you're new to Pilates or

Just returning from an injury, Wall Pilates is a wonderful place to get restarted.

Because it serves as a resistance, the Wall acts as a resistance training partner, which helps to tone and sculpt your muscles. If conducted properly, wall Pilates would birth the same outcome a traditional Pilates routine offers.

Benefits of Wall Pilates

This pattern of exercising is a great way to benefit from the numerous advantages Pilates offers:

Develops Core Strength

Locomotion is crucial to healthy living. However, so many of us are guilty of disobeying this simple health principle. The implication is that we would often develop weak core muscles. Pilates exercises help strengthen deep abdominal muscles, which resultantly affects our posture. The core includes the muscles at your back and sides; the Wall helps provide stability for your muscles which helps you focus on engaging your deep abdominal muscles. In this way, it is easier for the beginner.

Improves Endurance

Because the movements are slow and focused, Wall Pilates forces your muscles to be in motion for an extended period. This translates to increasing your muscular endurance levels. From lifting light weights to engaging in sporting activities, a healthy muscular endurance level is necessary for living. The resistance which the Wall provides also helps strengthen your muscles.

Flexibility

A Pilates exercise doesn't necessarily build your muscles. Instead, it focuses on lengthening the muscles. The Wall here provides support and stability and helps you deepen a stretch, improving flexibility.

Low Impact Activity

The average person dreads exercising because of the pain involved. Wall Pilates is a low-impact exercise; this means that it doesn't put much strain on your body. Other high-impact activities like running and jumping may cause a lot of wear and tear to the body, which may later lead to joint pains. The Wall here also serves as support, reducing the strain on the body. The exercise is suitable for persons with joint injuries.

Physical Rehabilitation

Pilates is famous for helping people recovering from pain and injury. The Wall in Pilates can support and stabilize this category of persons, helping them engage in some challenging positions.

Burns Calories

Wall Pilates is an excellent form of exercise that helps speed up metabolism by speeding up metabolism. This routine helps with losing weight by helping to burn calories. Research has it that the cardio and muscle strengthening exercises Pilates offer make it powerful for burning calories.

CHAPTER 2

UNDERSTANDING YOUR BODY TYPE

You put in all your effort; this time, you listened keenly to instructions, and after consuming all you thought there was about getting in shape, you thought you were certainly going to get it right this time. But you've viewed pictures of yourself from six months ago, and there's not a thing that has changed. Something must be missing! Doing the right exercise using the wrong body type is as good as doing 100% of nothing. As painful as that may sound, being oblivious to this fact can frustrate your weight loss plans.

Understanding your body type is extremely crucial to achieving your weight loss goals, so you'd want to find out where you fall within the different body types. We all have unique genetic or physiological designs that determine our body type, also known as somatype, and varied body types respond uniquely to different fitness programs. This makes it necessary to understand your body type.

Body types are essentially grouped into three categories: Ectomorphs, Endomorphs, and Mesomorphs. Ectomorphs appear thin and lean, having little muscles and body fat. People in this category usually find it difficult to gain weight. They have a fast metabolism which means that their calories burn faster. The kind of exercise suitable for Ectomorphs includes muscle-building exercises like weight training and squats.

Mesomorphs stand somewhere in the middle. This person has a fairly large bone structure and can be described as naturally athletic. A mesomorph finds it fairly easy to lose or gain weight.

Endomorphs, on the other hand, tend to have a higher percentage of body fat. They find it very easy to gain weight but have a slow metabolism rate, meaning they find it hard to lose weight. Focusing on exercises that help speed up metabolism is ideal for Endomorphs.

Individuals who find themselves in this category should focus more on both muscle-strengthening exercises and cardio practices to achieve their weight loss targets. Pilates provides these cardio and muscle-strengthening exercises, which help to boost metabolism and burn more calories.

Improving your Posture

So many ailments attack us only because we disobey some simple body rules. Back pain, neck pain, Joint arthritis, and even poor confidence level are all associated with bad posture. We would have many more people free from these conditions only if they maintained good posture.

We are not designed to live a sedentary life, but more often than not, we find ourselves glued to the computer screen, watching Television, tethered to our vehicles, and always on our mobile phones—all thanks to technology. If only we could find time to move about daily, we'd hardly complain about these issues. Sadly, bad posturing takes a toll on our bodies.

What is good posture, then? The definition of good posture is so varied between authors. Some say it's to have your spine straight or to stretch your shoulders as far back as possible, but good posture is attained when the spine, neck, and shoulders are all positioned in a way that allows you to be balanced.

Wall Pilates offers the opportunity to correct posture defects because Pilates teaches how to use your body efficiently. Consequently, weakened muscles would be strengthened, implying that correcting posture is a natural result of engaging in a Wall Pilates regime.

Setting Realistic Weight Loss Goals

A study by the University of Pennsylvania found that, on average, persons with overweight set a goal of losing 32% of their body mass. This is double or perhaps triple the amount needed for good health. Television and social media have made it so simple these days to make people feel awful about themselves. This has led to needless comparisons; everyone wants to be a Rihanna. It's not unlikely to find people setting unattainable goals in the name of improving their conditions. Setting unrealistic goals is a sure indication of failure.

Your weight loss goals can only be achieved if they are reasonable and attainable. The first step towards attaining your weight loss goals is making them realistic.

Set Mini Goals

To keep yourself energized toward your plan, consider making your goals bite-sized. For example, your goal may be to lose 10 pounds a month. Creating mini-goals helps give you the boost to continue with your weight loss plan. In keeping with your plan, make sure to track your improvement and always ensure you reward yourself for each eating and exercising habit fulfilled.

Think of setting process goals, such as working out all days in 2 months, rather than focusing on the weight or pounds to be lost. The trick is to look for activities that can be easily incorporated into your regular lifestyle. Rather than setting lofty goals that would almost always go nowhere, mini-goals are a great way to keep up with your weight loss goals.

Remember, slow and steady wins the race. Always remember that you are on this journey for the long haul, and celebrate every achievement in your weight loss plan. Whether it's losing 2 pounds a week or 10 a month, follow that consistently, each win provides the enthusiasm to keep moving.

The Science of Weight loss

So much is being peddled about this subject, but weight loss boils down to this one thing, the burning of calories. How many calories you burn determines how much weight you lose. We all require energy to function, and we get that energy from calories. Through foods such as carbohydrates, protein, and fat, energy is transmitted to your body, this fuel is gotten from the calories contained in them. This means that the more you consume these foods, the more calories you get. These calories in the body are then converted to the physical energy you'll need for your daily chores, but here's what happens: all the calories not converted are stored within your body as fat, and all of them remain in your body for as long as they are not used up.

To reduce these calories, you can do 2 things: cut down the intake of those foods with high calories or burn them off through physical activity. If you cut about 500 calories daily, you should lose about ½ to 1 pound weekly.

Leveraging Wall Pilates

A study carried out in 2012 revealed that participants who took Pilate routines burned more calories during their workouts and after more than those who did not participate. Wall Pilates is a wonderful form of exercise for weight loss as it helps boost metabolism and burn calories.

Research has found that combining cardio and muscle-strengthening exercises like Wall Pilates makes it perfect for burning calories. The speed of metabolism is what determines how many calories are burned in your body; this means that a higher metabolism rate ends in having more calories burned. Wall Pilates helps boost the metabolism rate, making it excellent for losing weight.

You should bear in mind that the number of calories burned in a Pilates' session depends on the intensity and how long the session lasts, this implies that conducting Wall Pilates exercises regularly would enhance the number of calories burned. Mainly on average, Wall Pilates can burn anywhere from 200 to 600 calories per hour. According to the American College of Sports Medicine, 150 to 250 moderate-intensity weekly exercises can stimulate weight loss. Two hundred fifty minutes of moderate-intensity exercise equals four to five weekly Wall Pilates sessions.

CHAPTER 3

BASIC WALL PILATES EXCERCISES

Welcome to the world of wall Pilates, where the simple act of standing against a wall can transform your body! Wall Pilates is an exceptionally effective way to tone your muscles, improve your posture, and enhance your flexibility without needing any equipment. Whether you're a beginner or an experienced Pilates' practitioner, wall exercises are a wonderful addition to your workout routine. So let's discover some of the best basic wall Pilates' exercises you can do to achieve a strong, healthy, and toned body.

Warm Up Exercises

Supported Roll Down

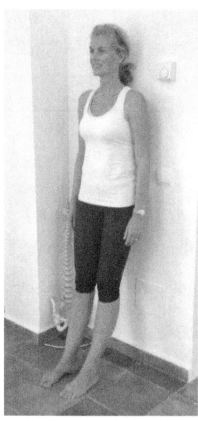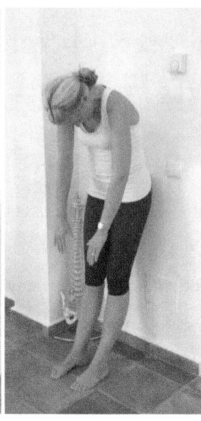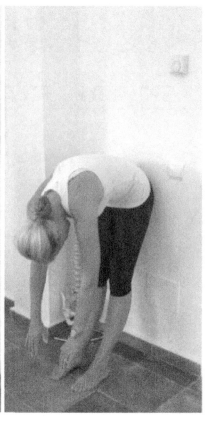

- Stand against a wall while retaining your back against the wall.

- Move back with your feet till they're six inches away.

- Fasten your core and hold your shoulders down, and feel relieved.

- As you breathe in, gradually roll your spine down the wall, vertebra by vertebra.

- Sense the muscles at your back stretching as you go down.

- Breathe out as you get to the bottom of the roll, holding your arms parallel to your sides.

- Hold for a set of breaths.

- Breathe in as you roll back up to the commencing position and redo this five more times.

Side Leg Swing

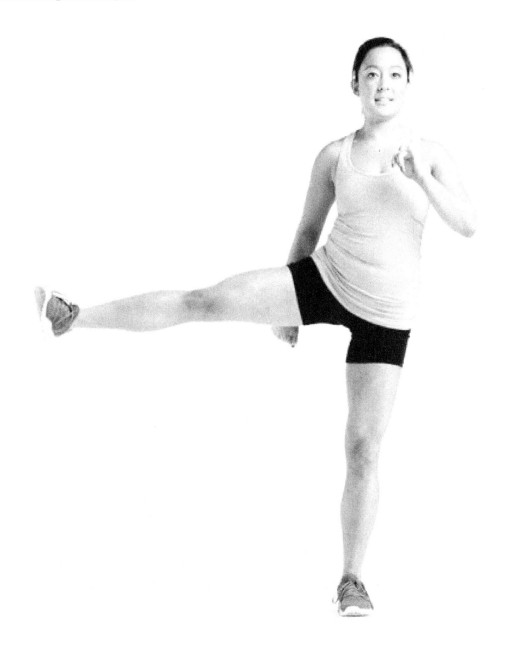

- Place one hand on the wall for support while standing next to it.

- Lift your outer leg so that your thigh is parallel to the ground.

- Make your pelvis level and look forward. Swing your leg out to the side and up as elevated as you can, maintaining your pelvis level.

- Switch the motion and swing your leg back to the commencing position.

- Redo on the other side.

Calf Stretch

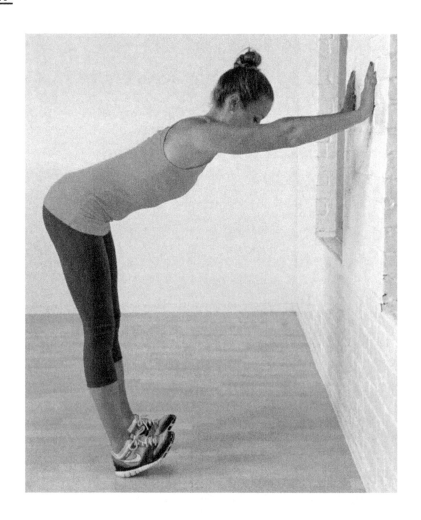

- Put your palms flat against the wall at shoulder altitude.

- Move your left leg back about two feet, maintaining your heel flat on the floor.

- Maintaining your left leg straight, stoop your right knee and lean into the wall till you sense a stretch in your left calf.

- Hold for a set of breaths.

- Free and repeat on the other side.

Wall Pilates Exercises For Weight Loss

You're already on your way to attaining your fitness desires; here are great Wall Pilates activities to put you right on track.

Wall plank

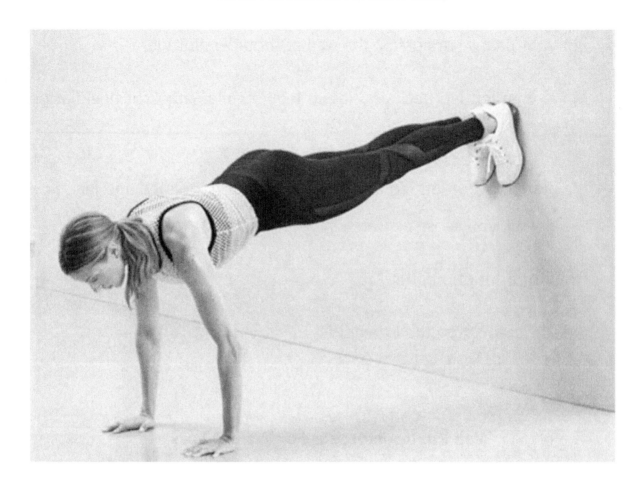

- Put your hands on the wall at shoulder height while facing the wall.

- Walk your feet back till your body forms a straight line from head to heels.

- Hold for 10-15 seconds, then slowly walk your feet back toward the wall. Repeat for 10-15 repetitions.

Wall Push-Ups

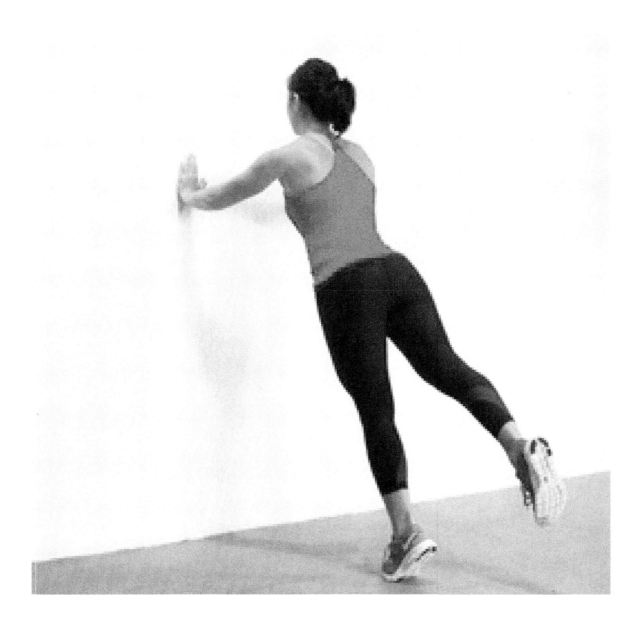

- Position your hands on the wall, a bit wider than shoulder-width apart, and walk your feet back till your body forms a diagonal line.

- Lower your chest towards the wall and push back up.

- Redo for 10 to 15 repetitions.

Wall Hundreds

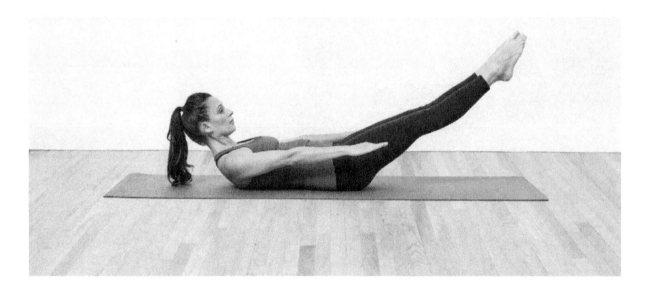

- Put your back down.

- Raise your two legs onto the tabletop and position both feet on the wall (your knees bent so your legs are at a right angle).

- Curl your head up, stretching out your arms long alongside your body, and palms put down.

- Push your arms up down as you breathe in for five counts (keeping palms down) and exhale for five counts (flipping to palms up).

- Redo this breathing style 10 times, still holding the position, changing palm direction for every five pumps.

Wall Sits

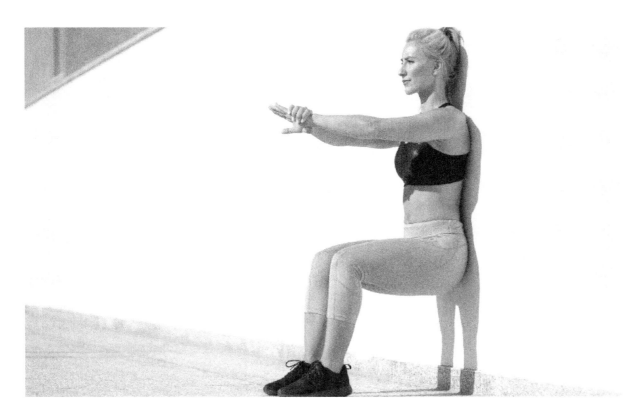

- Put your back against the wall while standing. Make sure your feet are about two feet away from the wall.

- Lower yourself gradually down the wall till your thighs are parallel to the floor.

- Maintain this position for 50 seconds or as long as you can hold on to it.

Wall Roll Down

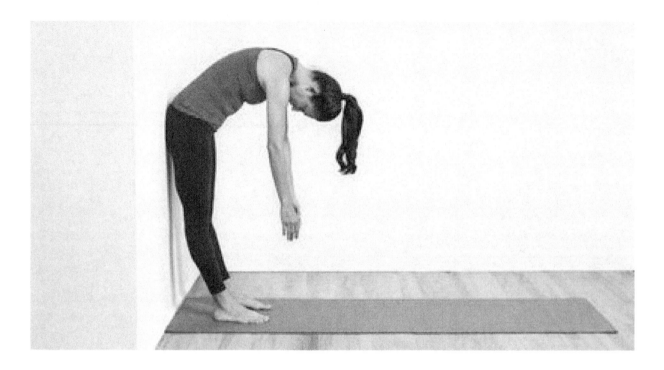

- While at your launching position, commence peeling away from the wall. Lower the chin towards your chest; next, start to pool away the shoulders. The arms hang loosely at your sides. Continue to pull the waist up and sense your low back shifting the wall away.

- Keep rolling down using the drawing in and up of the abs to let just one vertebra lose touch with the wall at a time. Keep at it until you get to a point where it is tough to do this. Your stomach continues to pull your mid-low back into the wall as the arms hang loose and free.

- Place each vertebra back against the wall as you rebuild your spine. Attempt to lengthen the spine as you carefully roll back up.

- Redo this 2-3 times, and on your last roll down, orbit your arms 4-8 times in each direction before rolling back up.

Wall Squats

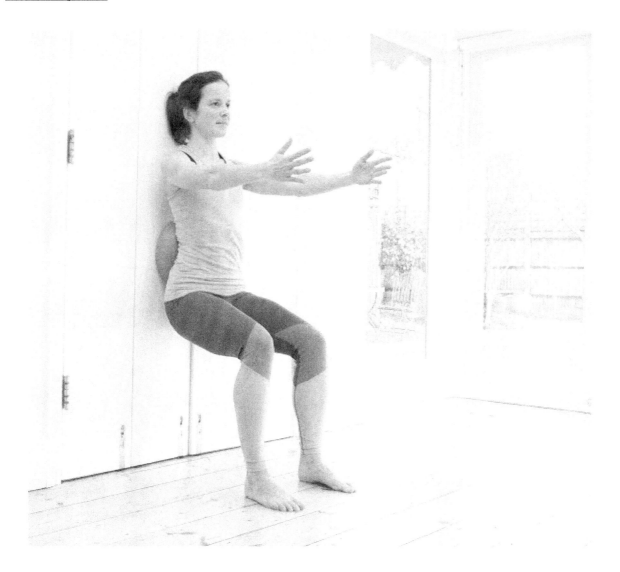

- Stand with your back against a wall and your feet hip-width apart.

- Slowly lower your body into a squat, pressing your back against the wall. Hold for 10-15 seconds, then slowly rise back up. Repeat for 10-15 repetitions.

- To increase the difficulty, you can hold weights in your hands.

- To vacate the wall, walk your feet back in, push back the palms of your hands against the wall, and walk forwards.

Wall Angels

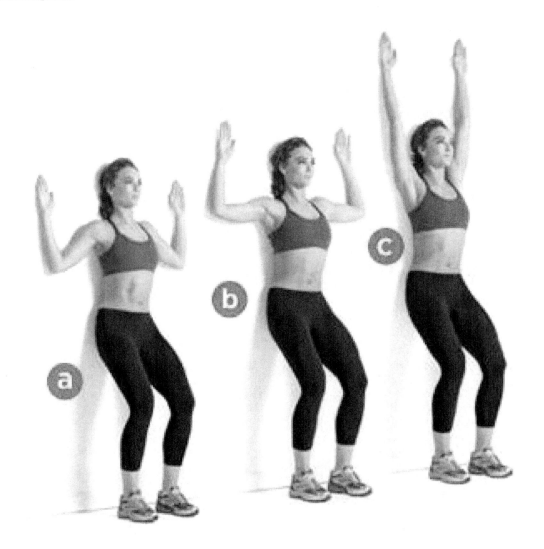

- Stand with your back against the wall, your feet hip-distance apart, your knees slightly bent, and your arms by your sides.

- Pull your belly button towards your spine, engage your core muscles, and press your lower back into the wall.

- Raise your arms to shoulder height, with your elbows bent at 90 degrees and your forearms parallel to the wall.

- Slowly slide your arms up the wall as high as you can while keeping your forearms and wrists in contact with the wall. Maintain a flat back and keep your shoulders away from your ears.

- Pause for a moment at the top of the movement, then slowly slide your arms back down to the starting position.

- Repeat for several repetitions.

Modification Tips for Varying Fitness Levels

The technique of using a wall for support in a Pilates exercise points towards the need for modification. The modification allows you to adapt an exercise depending on your body condition. Though a routine can be modified to make the exercise more challenging, especially if you're not very fit in specific areas of your body, here are tips to help you modify your routine.

Warm Up

There's no arguing the importance of a warm-up before properly moving into the main exercise. Taking your time to always warm up before the start of your routine would always go a long way to making your training effective. Starting with a warm-up would help prepare you for the full exercise.

The Weight of Your Arms

Just like your head, your arms are heavy. The farther they are from your body, the more demanding the exercise becomes; if you're considering taking a more challenging workout, using your arms as leverage is alright, but if you'll need support, you'd want to maintain your arms in a closed position.

Neck or Back Difficulties

If your injury has left you with any of these difficulties while exercising on your front or back, see that you leave your head down. Always see your head and neck as an extension of your spine. When on your belly, lift your head as an extension of your spine.

If you're just beginning Pilates, it could be better to focus on an easier variation of Wall Pilates; Wall Angels is a suitable exercise to try. If you notice any pain or discomfort in the course of the exercise, pause and reach out to your doctor or a certified Pilates instructor.

Form:

- Stand positioning your back against the wall, with your feet hip-distance apart, your knees slightly bent, and your arms placed by your sides.

- Pull your belly button towards your spine, engage your core muscles, and press your lower back into the wall.

- Lift your arms to shoulder height, with your elbows bent at 90 degrees and your forearms parallel to the wall.

- Gradually slide your arms up the wall as elevated as you can, keeping your forearms and wrists in contact with the wall. Place your shoulders down and away from your ears.

- Wait a moment at the top of the movement, then gradually slide your arms back down to the opening position.

- Repeat several times while maintaining proper form.

CHAPTER 4

ADVANCED WALL PILATES EXERCISES

I'm sure you're ready to take your Pilates practice to the next level! Maybe it's time to get to advanced wall Pilates exercises. These challenging and dynamic movements will push your body to new limits, testing your strength, endurance, and balance. From challenging variations of traditional Pilates exercises to innovative moves specifically designed for the wall, advanced wall Pilates will challenge you in ways you never imagined. Fret not, with dedication and practice; you can master these exercises and unlock a whole new level of physical and mental fitness. So let's dive in and explore some of the most challenging and rewarding advanced wall Pilates exercises to help you take your Pilates practice to the next level!

Wall Teaser:

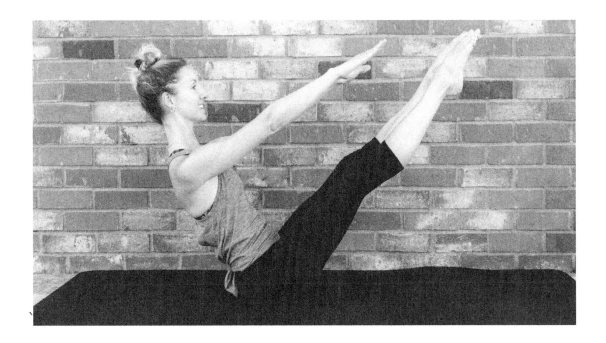

- Begin seated on the floor with your back against the wall; your legs extended in front of you.

- Engage your core and lift your legs to a tabletop position.

- Reach your arms straight up towards the ceiling.

- Begin to roll up, lifting your head and shoulders off the ground and reaching your arms forward.

- Keep rolling up until you are balancing on your sit bones with your legs and arms extended in front of you.

- Hold a few breaths, then roll back down to the starting position.

- Repeat for 5-10 repetitions.

Wall Bridge

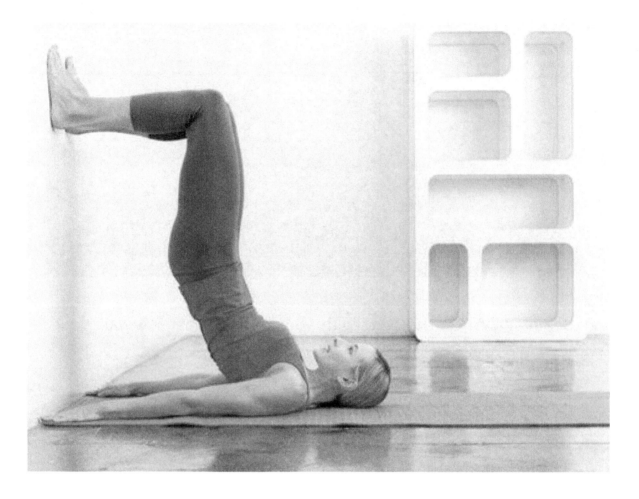

- Lie on your back with your feet flat against the wall, knees bent.

- Place your hands on the floor beside you and engage your core.

- Lift your hips up towards the ceiling, pushing through your feet against the wall.

- Hold a few breaths, then lower your hips back to the ground.

- Repeat for 10-15 repetitions.

Wall Arm Raise

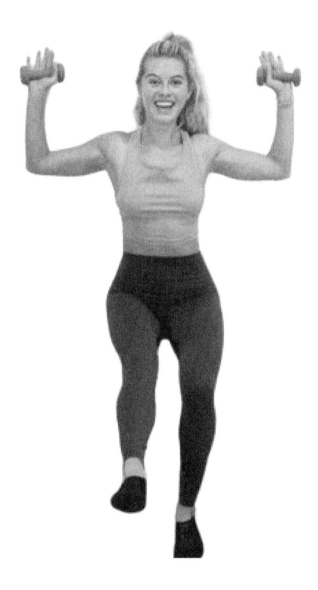

- With a light dumbbell in each hand, stand against the wall and bend your elbows to 90 degrees.

- Brace your core and gradually lift your arms till they are parallel to the floor.

- Hold a couple of breaths and lower your arms back to the launching position.

Wall Arm Circles

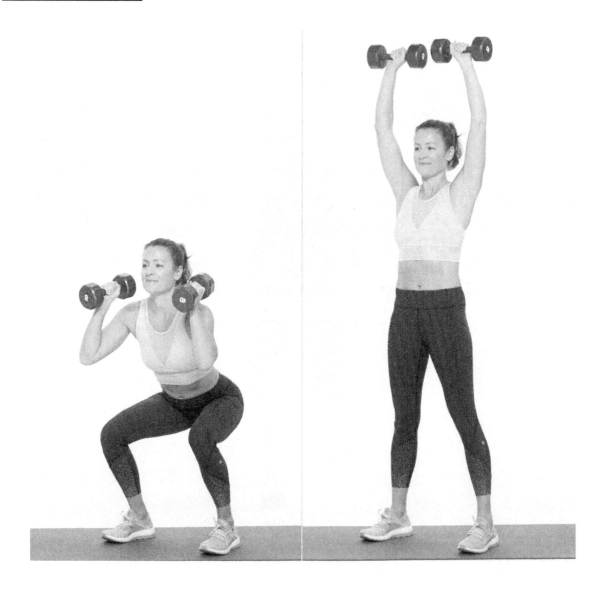

- With a light dumbbell in each hand, stand against the wall and bend your elbows to 90 degrees.

- Brace your core and gradually lift your arms till they are parallel to the ground.

- Still there, trace small circles in the air for about 30 seconds.

- Switch the direction of the circles and continue for another 30 seconds.

Scissors

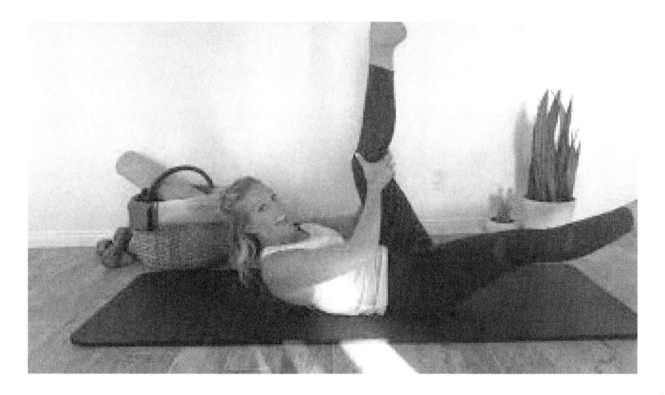

- With your bottom against the wall, lie down using your back and make sure your legs are straight up the wall.

- Still, with your legs against the wall, unlock them away from each other into a split as distant as you can go.

- Pull the legs back together. Complete 20 reps of this.

Forward Bend Back Leg Lift

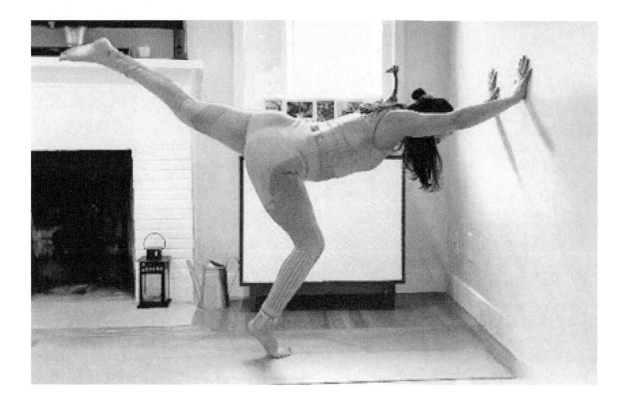

- Stand fronting the wall and bend to the front until your upper body is parallel to the floor.

- Press your palms against the wall while keeping your back flat. Lift your right leg behind you until it's parallel to the floor (or as elevated as possible).

- Bring the leg halfway down, approaching the floor, then raise it again. Complete 20 leg lifts on each side.

Forward Bend Side Leg Lift

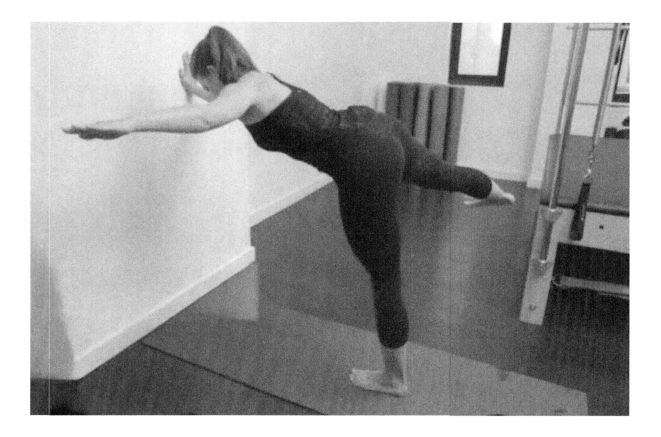

- Start in the same stance as the prior move, with your torso parallel to the floor and your hands pressing against the wall.

- Raise one leg to the side until it's parallel to the floor (or as tall as you can), maintaining your hips level.

- Complete 20 side leg lifts on each side.

Twist and Stretch

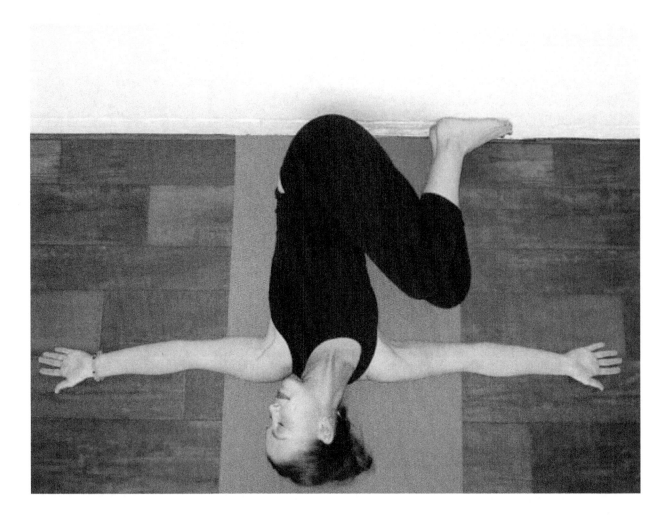

- Begin with your legs up the wall and your bottom attached to the wall.

- Draw your arms out to the side on the floor, perpendicular to your torso.

- Keep bending your knees until your feet are flat on the wall. Gradually walk both feet to your right until your right leg is laying on the floor, and you are in a deep spinal twist.

- Inhale and relax into the twist, maintaining your upper back against the floor.

- Keep for five slow deep breaths. Change sides by gradually walking your feet to the left.

- Redo this twice on each side.

Stretching Exercises

Spine Stretch

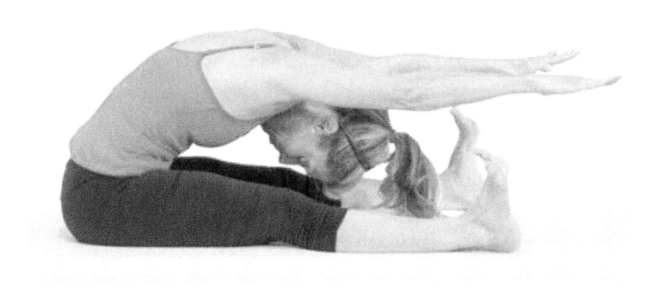

Spine stretch is a wonderful Pilates exercise for your back and hamstrings; still, it can provide a moment to center yourself before going on to more challenging exercises. Do it gently at the start of your routine, or use it for a more serious stretch later in your workout.

- Commence by sitting up tall, your back against a wall.

- Open your legs about shoulder distance apart and point your knees and toes toward the ceiling.

- Lift your arms right in front of you with palms facing down.

- Next, gradually roll your shoulders back as you inhale deeply into your belly.

- Then gradually curl your head down while pulling in your abs.

- Continue to roll forward toward your toes as if curling over a barrel.

- Next, inhale as you begin rolling back up the "wall," starting with your tailbone and ending with your head.

Saw

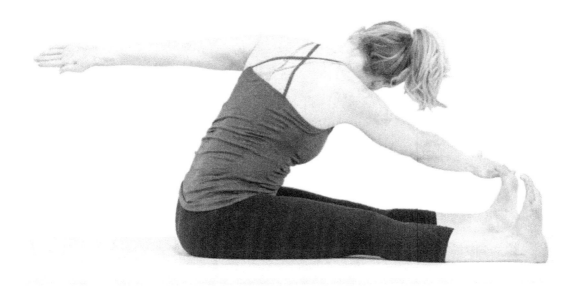

Saw is a great Pilates exercise for strength in your back extensors and stretching through the points of your fingers. It's also a good way to stretch your hamstrings.

- Sit down with your legs extended, feet flexed, and a little wider than your hips.

- Move to the sides and imagine you are trying to touch both room walls.

- Twisting toward your left leg, move your waist and arms as one unit.

- Maintain your pelvis on the mat.

- Slowly approach your left leg as you stretch back with your right arm; return with your left arm and then turn your palm up.

- Breathe as you reach forward, moving the top of your head toward your toes. Breathe in and sit up tall to get back to your commencing position. Redo this 3-5 times on each side.

Swan

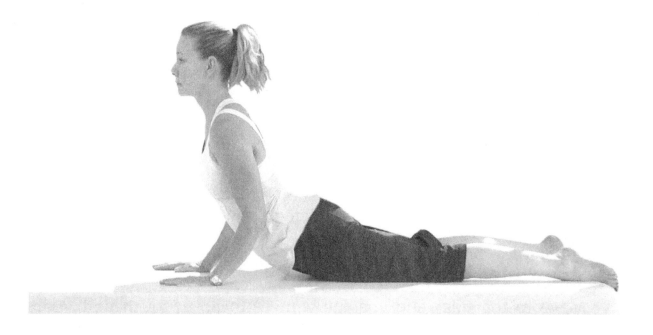

Swan Pilates can help you stretch the abdominals and hip flexors. Do more by adding a neck roll that will allow you to undergo a free range of motion when a strong core and stable upper body support your head and neck.

- Start by lying on the floor with your legs straight and putting your arms at your sides.

- Breathe out as you press into the floor using your hands and feet.

- Still in that position, move your tailbone close to the ceiling.

- Move to roll onto your upper back, releasing through the neck and shoulders.

- Wait for some seconds before breathing out and lowering yourself back down.

Mermaid Stretch

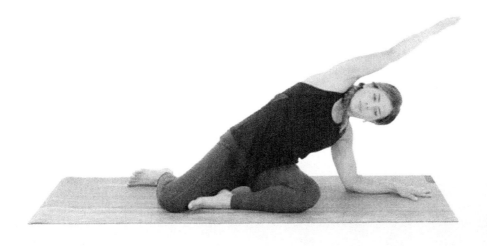

The Mermaid pose stretch can stretch and open the sides of your body, which may usually feel stiff in most people. When practicing this pose, ensure you keep the hips grounded as you take your arms up and over to feel the full stretch all the way through the center of your body.

- Start by sitting on your mat with your legs folded to one side and your feet close to your buttocks. Your knees should be bent, and your opposite hand should be placed on the mat behind your body to support your weight.

- Place your other hand on your head and lift your elbow towards the ceiling. This will help you lengthen the side of your body.

- Take a deep breath in, and as you exhale, side bend towards the floor, reaching your top elbow towards your bottom knee. Keep your shoulders and hips stacked, and avoid leaning forward or backward.

- Hold the stretch for a few breaths, feeling the lengthening sensation along the side of your body.

- Inhale as you lift back up to a tall sitting position.

CHAPTER 5

WALL PILATES ROUTINE FOR WEIGHT LOSS

I f you've been searching for a low-impact workout to help you lose weight, tone your muscles, and improve your overall fitness, wall Pilates is here for you. Specifically, in this chapter, we'll be focusing on a Wall Pilates routine for weight loss. Wall Pilates can be a great way to work out if you have limited space or if you're just starting out with Pilates. The wall provides support and stability, which can help you achieve proper form and alignment, reducing the risk of injury. Additionally, Wall Pilates is a full-body workout that engages multiple muscle groups, helping you burn calories and improve your cardiovascular health.

In this chapter, we'll share a Wall Pilates routine specifically designed for weight loss. We'll guide you through a series of exercises that will target your abs, legs, and arms while also helping you improve your posture and flexibility. We'll also provide modifications and variations for each exercise, so you can adjust the intensity of the workout to suit your fitness level.

So, get ready to sweat, tone, and sculpt your body with Wall Pilates!

Warm-Up Exercises

March in Place

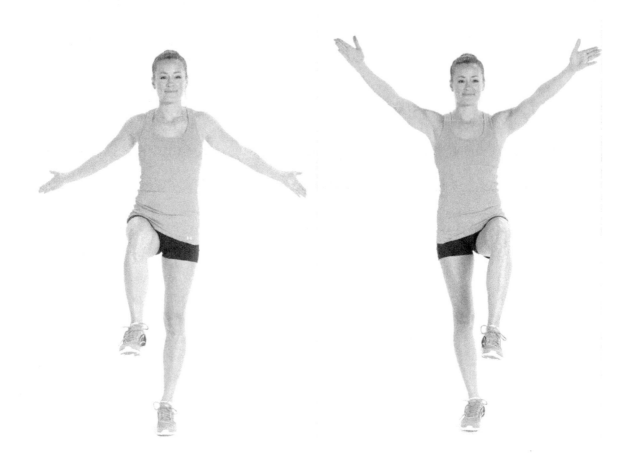

- Stand with your feet hip-width apart and march in place

- Raising your knees high.

- Continue for 1-2 minutes to elevate your heart rate and warm your legs.

Arm Circles

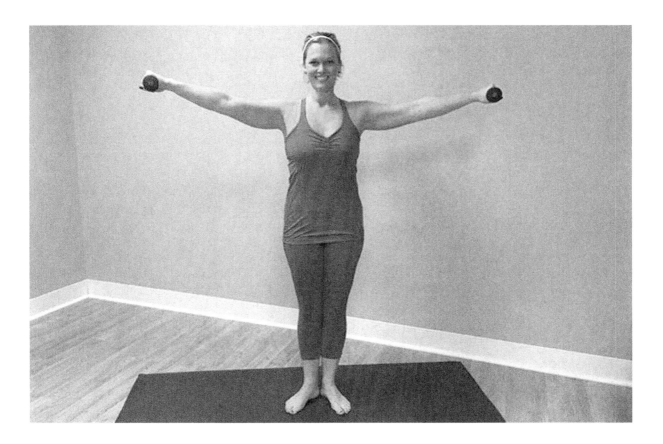

- Stand with your feet hip-width apart and raise your arms out to the sides, keeping them straight.
- Make small circles with your arms, slowly increasing the extent of the circles.
- Repeat 10-15 times in each direction.

Shoulder Rolls

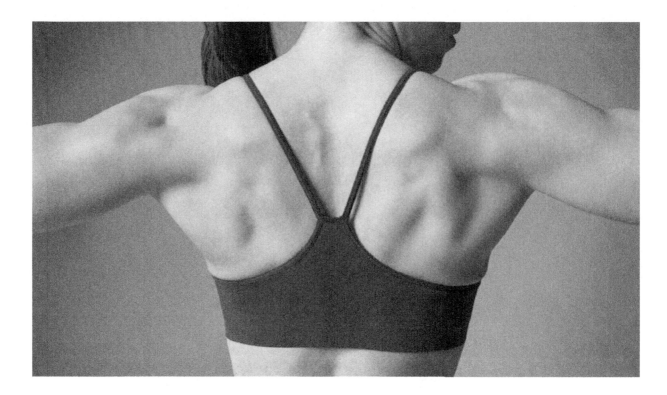

- Stand with your feet hip-width apart, your arms by your sides.

- Roll your shoulders forwards, then backwards.

- Do 10-15 repetitions for each direction.

<u>Neck Stretches</u>

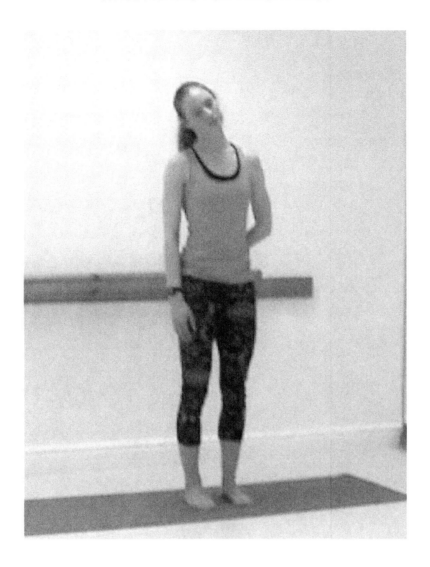

- Stand with your feet hip-width apart and your arms by your sides.

- Drop your chin towards your chest and hold for 10-15 seconds.

- Then, tilt your head towards the right, feeling a stretch in the left side of your neck.

- Hold for 10-15 seconds, then repeat on the other side.

Wall Pilates Routine to Burn Calories

Wall Squats

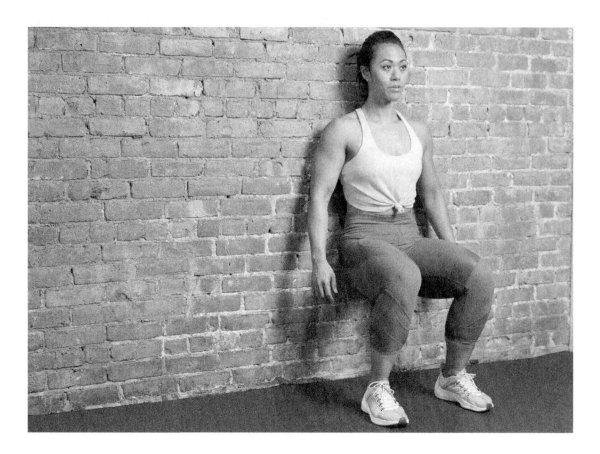

- Stand with your back against a wall and your feet hip-width apart.

- Gradually lower your body into a squat, keeping your back pressed against the wall.

- Hold for about 10-15 seconds,

- Then gradually rise back up. Redo for 10-15 repetitions. To increase the difficulty, you can hold weights in your hands.

Wall Push-Ups

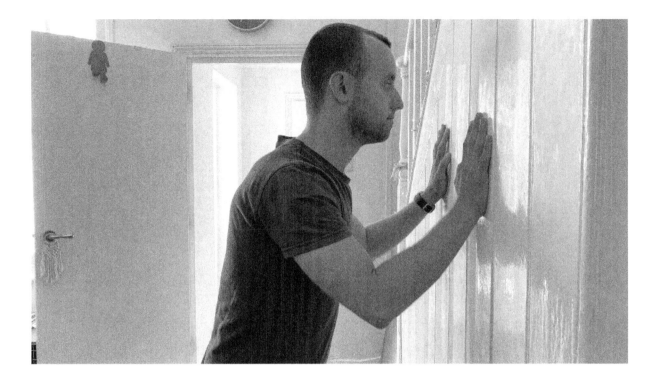

- Stand facing a wall with your arms lengthened in front of you and your hands flat against the wall.

- Gradually bend your elbows and lower your body towards the wall, maintaining your back straight.

- Push back up to the opening position. Repeat for 10-15 repetitions. You can move your feet a distance away from the wall to increase the difficulty.

Wall Sit With Leg Lifts

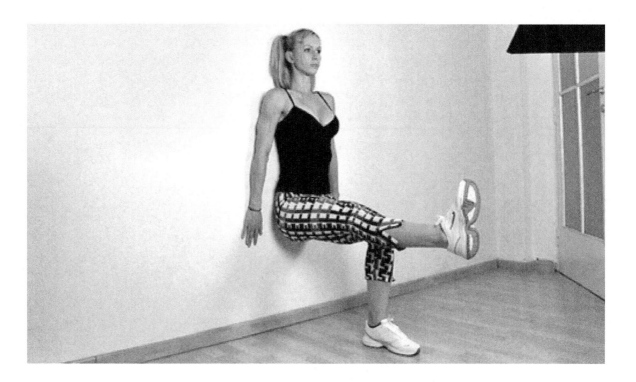

- Stand with your back against a wall, your feet hip-width apart.

- Lower down into a wall sit, with your thighs parallel to the floor.

- Hold for 10-15 seconds, then lift your right leg and hold for 10-15 seconds.

- Lower your leg and redo on the left side. Redo for about 10-15 repetitions for each leg. To intensify, you can carry weights in your hands or do a single-leg wall.

Wall Plank

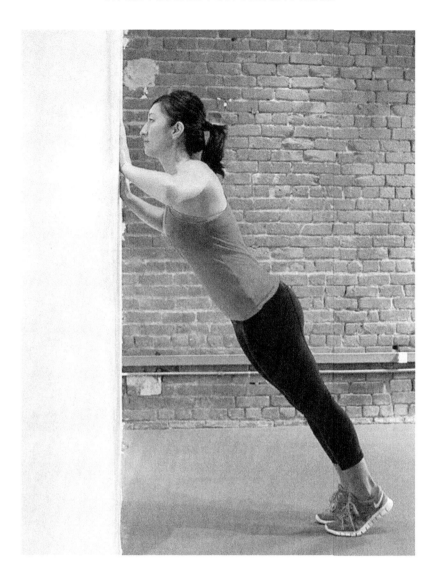

Stand facing a wall and put your hands on the wall at shoulder height.

Walk your feet back till your body forms a straight line from head to heels. Hold for about 10-15 seconds, then gradually walk your feet back towards the wall. Redo for 10-15 repetitions. To intensify, you can hold the plank for longer or move your hands a distant away from the wall.

Wall Ab Curls

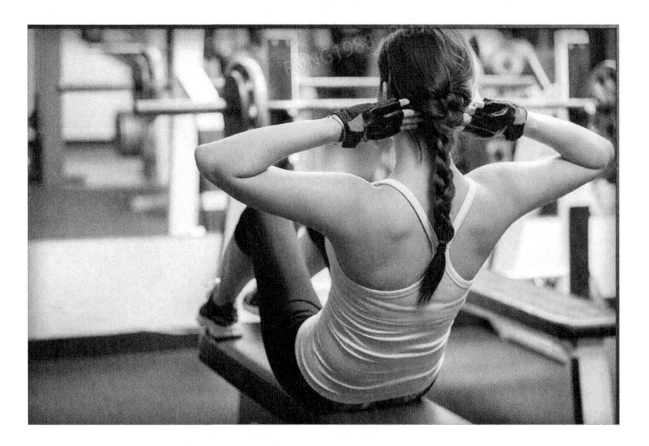

- Sit on the ground with your back placed against the wall and your knees bent.

- Position your hands behind your head and raise your shoulders off the ground, curling your torso towards your knees.

- Lower back down and redo 10-15 times.

- To make it more challenging, you can grip a weight in your hands or straighten your legs.

Cool down

Hamstring Stretch

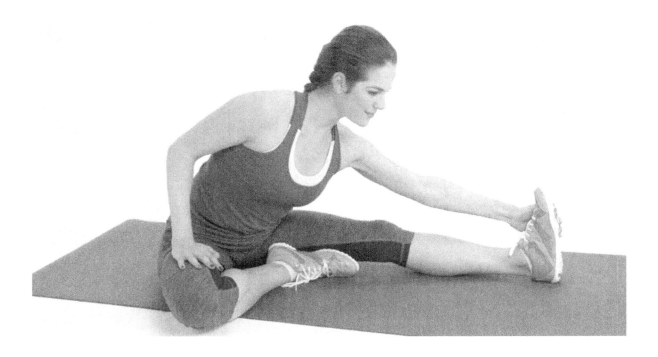

- Sit on the floor with your legs extended straight out in front of you.

- Reach forward attempting to touch your toes, feeling a stretch in the back of your legs.

- Hold for about 10-15 seconds.

Quad Stretch

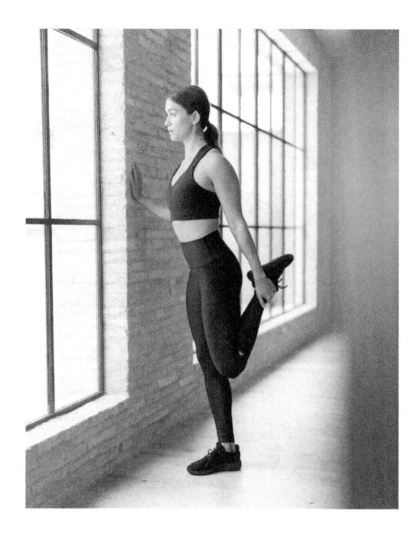

- Stand looking at the wall and put your left hand on the wall for support.

- Bend your right knee and grasp your ankle using your right hand, feeling a stretch in the front of your thigh.

- Hold for 10-15 seconds, then redo for the other side.

Shoulder Stretch

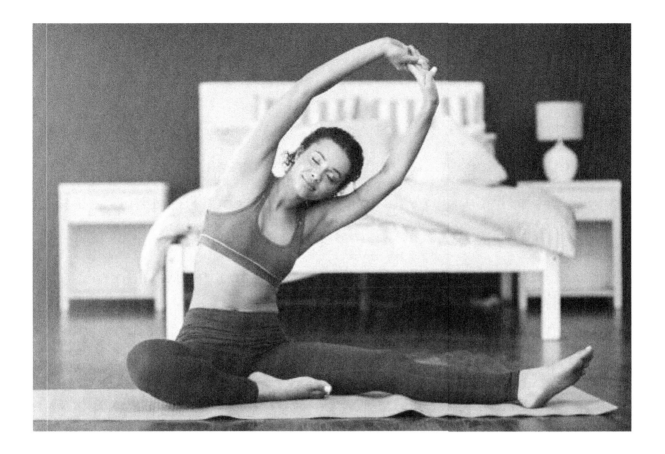

- Stand with your feet hip-width apart and clasp your hands behind your back.

- Raise your hands up.

Proper Form and Technique

To get the most out of any Pilates' routine, merely practicing the exercise is not enough. You'd have to engage the proper form and technique as they're highly crucial in Pilates' exercises. First, using the right form and technique helps you with effectiveness. Through using the right technique and form you're better able to engage the right muscles effectively and most likely to get the results you want.

Practicing this way also helps you prevent injury. By using the right alignment and engaging the right muscles, you're less likely to experience joint injuries or injuries to your joints and ligaments. Furthermore, it helps you develop a mind-body connection. By focusing on the right muscles and alignment, you will become aware of your body and the way it moves.

Truth is: using proper form and techniques generally rubs off on your life; by practicing this, you become more mindful and aware of your body and what you do to it. The most vital reason you'd have to engage proper form and technique is that that's the way you can make your wall Pilates routine get you the results you want.

Incorporating Wall Pilates into Your lifestyle

This is a good point to remind you that you're what you constantly do. Integrating Wall Pilates into your lifestyle can be a terrific way to attain your weight loss goals. Here are some methods to fix wall Pilates into your daily life.

Make it Part of Your Schedule.

You already have your day all planned; there's time for sleeping and meeting up with a friend. It's time to add Wall Pilates to that list, just as you would for any other meeting or schedule. Add Wall Pilates to your calendar.

Get a Friend

Having a Wall Pilates buddy is a great way to keep your motivation and make the practice enjoyable. With your friend, you can always get the encouragement to keep up with your Wall Pilates practice. So, get a workout buddy for your wall Pilates practice.

Start Small

If you're just starting out, you should be easy on yourself and don't think of lofty routines that may be unattainable for the time. Instead, start with a shorter routine; you can move to longer sessions as time progresses.

Pay Attention to Your Body

As zealous as you are toward getting that perfect body shape. Do not try to push yourself beyond limits. If a practice appears too hard on you, consider modifying it. Also, make sure to always take breaks when necessary.

As you begin to incorporate this gentle but effective exercise into your lifestyle, you are sure to hit your target of shedding those pounds.

Incorporating Wall Pilates into Your Daily Routine

You are what you do daily! Take your weight loss goals a step further by looking for ways to integrate wall Pilates into your daily routine. That way, you're sure of reaping the benefits that come with this practice.

Often, it may appear this exercise is unable to fit into your daily schedule, but if you'll look closely, there's always a way to compress time. For example, most of us spend time boiling a quick cuppa in the morning. You can spend those few minutes doing a Wall roll-down. There are several times like this in your day that you can utilize for your Pilates practice; you'd only have to look closely.

Building a Workout Routine

There are many ways to carry on with your fitness goals, and following a set routine is cool, but learning how to create a workout routine for yourself is one of the promising ways to support your weight loss plans.

In building a routine, you should consider the vital elements which make up an effective workout routine. An ideal workout routine should include the following:

Plan

Exercising off the top of your head may work sometimes, but planning your workout session is recommended for achieving the results you want. In making your routine, think about your weight loss goals; for example, what's your energy level? Are there key areas of your body you'd like to work on? These questions would help you tailor your workout properly.

Warm-up

An ideal routine must contain a beginning, middle, and end. Before you start properly, warming up is necessary to loosen up the muscles and tone your body in preparation for the main exercise. These exercises can, however, be modifications of those you'd practice later on in your workout.

Range and Rotation

Once you're done warming up, it's time to engage in more demanding exercises. Workouts that turn and twist your body can be added now. Before practicing exercises that twist your spine, make sure you've done a proper warm-up.

Modifications

The idea of modifying is not to defeat the purpose of the exercise. By doing this, you still maintain the reason for the exercise but make it either easier or harder to suit your specific needs; when building your routine, you may consider modifying it.

Finish Well

How you end matters a lot, you'd want to do this consciously. Think of exercises that can transit you properly. Bring the pace down, draw your attention inward, and regulate your breath. A Pilates exercise focuses on readying your body for everyday life and concludes by checking how much you've done.

Staying Motivated

The science of weight loss in some way is commitment. No matter how well-intentioned you are, without commitment, it's near impossible that you'd get results, but how can you be committed without staying motivated? Here are some tips to help you stay motivated.

Create the Perfect Space

So much about what we do relates to where we do it; there is an invisible nexus between where we stay and what we get. Having the perfect space for your Wall Pilates training may just do the magic for you. It doesn't have to be a stadium. It may just be a place where you are more relaxed, with the nicest view or anything else.

Pay for Your Sessions

Though Wall Pilates provides an inexpensive exercise method, you might just find it beneficial to commit yourself by paying even for your at-home workouts. It doesn't have to be so much. The whole idea is just to keep you committed; this can be done by having a virtual instructor.

Make it an Appointment.

It's so easy to give in to distractions, especially when we're under no control. Put your workout session on a schedule, make it a commitment, and set alarms for your workout, this way you're signaling to your body that this is very crucial and it's not something you'd want to compromise.

CHAPTER 6

NUTRITION FOR WEIGHT LOSS

Working out is a fantastic way to burn off calories which end up being stored as fats in our bodies. But that's only one way! A second technique is to stop these calories from entering in the first place. While working out is a great way to help drop some pounds, combining this practice with proper eating habits is crucial for weight loss.

The key to healthy and sustainable weight loss lies in proper nutrition, as a balanced and nutritious diet would not only help you shed unwanted pounds but also improve your overall health and well-being. In this chapter, we'll explore the power of nutrition for weight loss and discuss the foods that can help you reach your goals. From the importance of protein and fiber to the usefulness of whole foods and healthy fats, we'll supply you with the tools you need to make smart nutritional choices and achieve lasting weight loss. It's also very important to note that If you practice these Wall Pilates techniques but keep on with your negative eating habits, you are unlikely to notice any significant changes. So, let's dive in and discover how proper nutrition can help you achieve your weight loss goals for good!

Healthy Eating Habits to Complement Your Wall Pilates Routine.

Starting a weight loss plan is not a license to destroy your body. Calories are still very essential for the development of your body, but the most vital factor in weight loss is a negative calorie balance. This means that you'll need to burn off more calories than you take into your body.

If you're looking to reduce your weight, most of your nutrition should come from vegetables and grain products, which supply many nutrients to the body. With this, the body doesn't suffer while trying to reduce calories.

Reduce Refined Carbohydrates

The interesting thing about cutting down on carbohydrates is that it helps keep your hunger level down, which causes you not to take high-calorie foods.

Instead, you should consider taking low carbs or taking more complex carbs like whole grains. Reduce the intake of starch and sugars. By taking complex carbs, things get better because consuming complex carbs such as whole grains contains high fiber, which helps the food digest better.

Vegetables, Proteins

You'd want to consider having a lot of vegetables on your plate as they contain a lot of nutrients without transmitting so many calories. However, you should be cautious of some vegetables, like sweet potatoes, which are high in carbs. Instead, try out, broccoli, spinach, and tomatoes.

Taking in some proteins may be important as this may help reduce your craving for junk and snacking. Plant-based proteins like legumes and tofu are a good way to go.

Take Fats in Moderation

Fats are a vital source of energy for your body. However, if you're on a weight loss plan, you'd have to focus on taking low-fat meals. Healthy fats like fish, avocado, and flax oil are still essential for your body, however.

Proper Hydration

There's truly no fat burning in the absence of water. If you're looking to lose weight, you should try so much to stay hydrated; consider taking at least 1.5 to 2 liters of water every day, and make sure to avoid alcohol and unnecessary sugars as they are full of needless calories.

Seven-Day Meal Plan For Weight Loss

This is a sample 7-day meal plan to assist in your weight loss goals:

Monday:

Breakfast: Greek yogurt with berries and a sprinkle of granola.

Snack: Apple slices with almond butter.

Lunch: Mixed greens, cherry tomatoes, cucumbers, and balsamic vinaigrette with grilled chicken salad.

Snack: Baby carrots with hummus.

Dinner: Brown rice and baked salmon with roasted broccoli.

Tuesday:

Breakfast: Spinach and mushroom omelet with whole wheat toast.

Snack: A handful of almonds.

Lunch: Turkey and avocado sandwich with lettuce and tomato on whole wheat bread.

Snack: Banana with peanut butter.

Dinner: Quinoa bowl with black beans, corn, avocado, and salsa.

Wednesday:

Breakfast: Smoothie made with spinach, banana, almond milk, and protein powder.

Snack: Greek yogurt with a drizzle of honey.

Lunch: Grilled chicken with sweet potato and green beans.

Snack: Fresh berries.

Dinner: Grilled shrimp with roasted Brussels sprouts and quinoa.

Thursday:

Breakfast: Whole grain cereal with almond milk and berries.

Snack: Baby carrots with tzatziki sauce.

Lunch: Tuna salad with mixed greens and cherry tomatoes.

Snack: Edamame.

Dinner: Chicken stir-fry with mixed vegetables and brown rice.

Friday:

Breakfast: Scrambled eggs with spinach and whole wheat toast.

Snack: A handful of grapes.

Lunch: Grilled chicken Caesar salad.

Snack: Roasted chickpeas.

Dinner: Baked sweet potato topped with black beans, salsa, and avocado.

Saturday:

Breakfast: Greek yogurt with sliced banana and honey.

Snack: A small apple.

Lunch: Turkey chili with a side salad.

Snack: Hummus with cucumber slices.

Dinner: Baked chicken with roasted carrots and quinoa.

Sunday:

Breakfast: Smoothie made with mixed berries, Greek yogurt, and almond milk.

Snack: A small orange.

Lunch: Grilled salmon with roasted asparagus and brown rice.

Snack: Baby carrots with guacamole.

Dinner: Baked cod with mixed vegetables and quinoa.

Remember, this is only a sample. To make the most of your weight loss goals, consult a registered dietitian or health care professional to create a personalized meal plan that fits your unique needs.

CHAPTER 7

LIFESTYLE TIPS FOR WEIGHT LOSS

Do you find it difficult to stick to your weight loss plan despite giving it your best try? Then it's time to learn something new! The key to sustainable weight loss lies in making healthy lifestyle changes that you can maintain long-term. By adopting healthy habits that fit seamlessly into your daily routine, you can attain your weight loss goals and feel your best. In this chapter, we'll explore lifestyle tips for weight loss that go beyond just counting calories. From simple changes you can make to your diet to simple ways to incorporate exercise into your day. These tips will help you create a healthier, happier, more sustainable lifestyle. So let's move on to discover the lifestyle changes that can help you attain your weight loss goals!

Eat Regularly

As counterintuitive as this may sound, proper feeding is important for your weight loss goals. Eating regularly discourages sudden hunger and unbridled food cravings that may cause you to consume unnecessary calories. So, you'd want to make it a habit to take your meals when you should have them. This doesn't imply overeating, and you must still stick with taking low-calorie foods.

Getting Adequate Sleep

Whenever your body is asleep, your metabolism is running at full throttle. This implies that insufficient sleep would almost always leads to weight gain because it affects the speed of metabolism. As a lifestyle, ensure to always get good enough sleep. Again, this is not a license for sleeping excessively, as this can lead to negative consequences for your body.

Avoid Stress

Experiencing stressful situations appears to be an inevitable part of everyday living. However, you must try as much as possible to avoid stress-producing situations. This is because whenever you're stressed, the body releases a hormone known as cortisol which inhibits the burning of fat in your body. Always look for ways to avoid stress; for example, taking breaks and relaxing can go a long way.

Walk More Often

Stop burning gas, start burning calories! It's been said that each extra hour you spend driving is connected with a six percent increase in obesity. Almost all the time, we are driving out in our automobiles. You must have learned that we are not designed for a sedentary lifestyle. There's so much walking more often would do. Whenever you have just a few miles, try your legs instead. This minor change would mean a lot for your body.

Maintain a Food Journal

Putting pen to paper creates awareness. Make a habit of journaling all that you eat in a day; this would help you track all that you've taken for the day. That would help show where you're lacking, such as how much junk food you ate for the day. By knowing this, you can always improve your eating habit.

Restrict Processed Foods

Most packaged foods are high in sugar, fat, and sodium. These contents are opposed to weight loss plans, so you'd do well to limit your intake of these products. It may not be easy starting, but you can start by making daily targets of reducing by just a product per day until you're strong enough to stop.

Keeping up With Your Plan

As with new year's resolutions, it's easy to say: this year, I'd make sure to practice wall Pilates every day, I'd avoid taking high-carb foods, or I'm getting processed foods off my list! Good a thing. But the majority of even well-intentioned individuals end up giving up on their plans.

Here's the thing, it's not starting these practices that would get you into that perfect body; it's being consistent with the routine. If you've tried your best with previous exercises but seem to always fall out, here are some key tips to help keep you motivated and consistent.

Intrinsic Motivation

What's your reason for working out? Is it pressure from friends, getting the approval of your colleagues, or maybe appearing nicely for the next event? The truth is: it's harder to keep with your routine when motivation doesn't come from within. The right attitude is to think about the personal fulfillment you'd get from improving yourself.

Talk Positively

Remember that this is a journey, and you may not get it all correct every day. If you miss a day or two, don't speak negatively; pat yourself on the back and keep going. Don't ever say the routine is complex; instead, you may say it's challenging.

Practice Things You Enjoy

The best way to build momentum is to start with things you already enjoy. You should start by focusing on activities and diets that you already fancy. Try searching for alterations that make your favorite dish lower in calories. Or still, at some point, have your choice dish as a side serving.

Make Your Workout Fun

Resist the possibility of making workout time the worst time of your day; instead, incorporate fun activities into your workout time. For example, listening to your favorite playlist. Rather than being boring, workout time should be a time you'd look forward to every day; it all depends on you.

Look For a Weight Loss Partner

Regardless of where they are used, partnerships are always great. Having a weight loss companion can help keep you consistent since it's fun to train together. And again, your partner can always hold you accountable for your workout routine.

Commitment

Wall Pilates is an incredible way to achieve weight loss goals, but consistency is key, like any fitness routine. More than starting, commitment and consistency to your routine would ultimately lead you to achieve your weight loss goals. There would be a time when the changes wouldn't be visible. During these times, it is your commitment that counts. To understate commitment is to live in denial; here are some tips to help you stay committed.

Set realistic goals: Set achievable goals that you can work towards, such as performing a certain number of repetitions of a specific exercise. It's hard to stay committed to a lofty and unrealistic goal.

Mix it up: Incorporate a variety of wall Pilates exercises into your routine to keep things interesting and prevent boredom; this way, you're energized to continue your routine.

Track your progress: Try to keep track of your progress by taking measurements or snapshots. Seeing your progress can be a powerful motivator to help you keep on with your routine.

Change is constantly happening. Each day you show up is each time you decide to discipline yourself. Remember, it is not the final hit that brings down the wall; it is cumulative of all those efforts.

So, don't stop showing up. Keep at your routine. You'd soon find that you are a changed person.

CONCLUSION

Congratulations on completing this book on Wall Pilates for weight loss! By now, you have learned about the benefits of wall Pilates exercises, how to create a routine, and the importance of proper nutrition. You have also discovered tips to help you stay committed to your practice in achieving your weight loss goals. Coming this far is a great indicator that you'd ultimately get into that perfect body. Wall Pilates is indeed effective for weight loss, as you have learned.

The vast majority of people think of Pilates as a gentle, soft, and peaceful form of exercise. Since most of us hold the idea that toughness equals effectiveness, it is no surprise that most people would hardly agree that there's a connection between weight loss and Pilates. This book challenges that narrative. With the techniques presented in this book, weight loss gets even easier, as the only equipment needed for this practice is a wall.

Wall Pilates may just be your access to that dream lean and thin body. This exercise which focuses on lengthening, strengthening and toning the whole body, is a great practice for weight loss. In fact, a study conducted by the Guangzhou University of Chinese Medicine found that compared to other exercises, this exercise leads to a significant decrease in body weight, body mass weight (BMI), and body fat percentage of overweight people.

Importantly, wall Pilates is an exercise that seeks to improve your calorie balance. The exercises allow you to burn off more calories than you consume, resulting in weight loss.

The exercises practiced in wall Pilates emphasize fluidity, which means that learners transition from one exercise to another, having only minimal time for rest. This very act makes it effective for burning off calories. When combined with proper dieting, practicing wall Pilates will surely get you to your weight loss dreamland. There are no two ways about it; getting proper nutrition is also an invaluable part of the weight loss plan.

Remember that consistency and patience are key when it comes to any fitness routine, so rather than thinking of a quick fix, consider setting more sustainable and achievable goals. As you continue to practice, you may find that your body becomes stronger, more flexible, and better balanced. Keep going! With the right nutrition, wall Pilates would support your efforts to achieve lasting weight loss.

By incorporating wall Pilates into your daily routine, you can enhance your overall health and well-being. So, grab your mat and head to the wall, and let Wall Pilates become a staple in your fitness journey. Surely, with dedication and commitment, you'd achieve your weight loss goals to enjoy a healthier, happier, and more balanced life.

OTHER BOOKS BY THE AUTHOR

2-MINS WALL PILATES FOR SENIORS

Scan below to get a COPY now

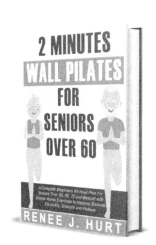 

2 MINUTES HOME WORKOUTS FOR SENIORS OVER 50

Scan below to get a COPY now

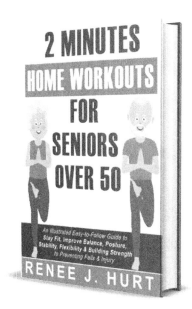 

FEEDBACK & APPRECIATION

Thank you for purchasing our book!

If you enjoyed this book, please consider dropping us a REVIEW.

It takes 5 seconds and helps small publishing businesses like ours thrive.

Please Scan below to drop your Review

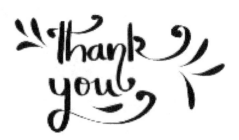

Printed in Great Britain
by Amazon

23863337R00057